# Osteoporosis Diet Cookbook

## Prevent and Treat Your Bones with Delicious Recipes

### Dr Olivia Tastewell

<h1 style="text-align:center">Copyright © 2024 by Dr  Olivia Tastewell</h1>



Kindly scan the barcode below to reach out to the author and have access to more of our books.

# TABLE OF CONTENTS

# Introduction

CONSIDER YOURSELF GOING DOWN the street on a beautiful day when you slip and fall. You know you've fractured your wrist after feeling a severe ache in it. What caused this to happen? You're not old, you're not sick, and you're not frail. You are one of millions of Americans who suffer from osteoporosis, a disorder that causes your bones to become weak and brittle. Osteoporosis is a silent illness that affects both men and women, however, it is more prevalent after menopause. It is believed that 10 million Americans have osteoporosis, and another 44 million have inadequate bone density, putting them at risk of fracture. Osteoporosis puts half of all persons 50 and older in danger of fracturing a bone. Chronic pain, paralysis, loss of independence, and even death can all result from osteoporosis.

However, there is some good news. A bone-friendly diet and lifestyle can help you avoid and cure osteoporosis. You may strengthen your bones and minimize your risk of fractures by consuming meals high in calcium, vitamin D, protein, and other minerals. You may also enhance your bone health by undertaking weight-bearing and muscle-strengthening activities regularly, avoiding smoking and excessive alcohol use, and taking medicines as directed by your doctor. This cookbook has 30 tasty and simple breakfast, lunch, and supper meals that will feed your bones and body. You will learn how to select and cook calcium-rich meals such as dairy products, seafood, leafy greens, and fortified foods. You'll also learn how to incorporate vitamin D-rich foods like fatty fish, eggs, mushrooms, and fortified foods into your diet. You'll also learn how to balance your protein, magnesium, potassium, vitamin C, vitamin K, and other nutrients needed for bone health. This cookbook is for you if you suffer from osteoporosis, have low bone density, or just want to avoid bone loss. It will assist you in maintaining a balanced and enjoyable diet that will aid your bones and general well-being. So, what are you holding out for? Let's put on our aprons and start cooking!

# Breakfast Recipes

## Red Marvel Smoothie

Ingredients:

- 1 cup raspberries (fresh or frozen)
- 1/2 cup blueberries (fresh or frozen)
- 1/4 cup prunes, chopped
- 1 tablespoon oats
- 1 cup cranberry juice
- 1 teaspoon lemon juice
- 1/2 cup nonfat Greek yogurt

Nutritional Information (per serving):

- Calories: 250
- Fat: 3g (1g saturated)
- Carbs: 30g (4g fiber)
- Protein: 12g
- Calcium: 300mg (30% DV)

Serving size: 1 smoothie

Cooking time: 5 minutes

**Instructions:**

1. In a blender, combine all of the ingredients and mix until smooth.
2. Enjoy immediately for a refreshing and nutrient-rich breakfast.

Label: Calcium-rich, high in antioxidants, fiber-packed, vegan (omit yogurt for fully vegan).

# Citrus Berry Smoothie

**Ingredients:**

- 1 cup mixed berries (fresh or frozen)
- 1 orange, peeled and segmented
- 1/2 cup nonfat Greek yogurt
- 1/4 cup unsweetened almond milk
- 1 tablespoon chia seeds
- 1/2 teaspoon honey (optional)

**Nutritional Information (per serving):**

- Calories: 200
- Fat: 3g (1g saturated)
- Carbs: 25g (4g fiber)
- Protein: 15g
- Calcium: 200mg (20% DV)

Serving size: 1 smoothie

Cooking time: 5 minutes

**Instructions:**

1. In a blender, combine all of the ingredients and mix until smooth.
2. Add honey to taste if desired.
3. Enjoy immediately for a vitamin-packed and protein-rich breakfast.

Label: High in vitamin C, a good source of calcium, dairy-free option (use plant-based yogurt).

# Almond Butter and Banana Toast

Ingredients:

- 1 slice of whole-wheat bread
- 1/4 cup mashed ripe banana
- 2 tablespoons almond butter
- 1/4 cup sliced strawberries (optional)
- Pinch of cinnamon (optional)

Nutritional Information (per serving):

- Calories: 250
- Fat: 10g (2g saturated)
- Carbs: 30g (4g fiber)
- Protein: 8g
- Calcium: 30mg (3% DV)

Serving size: 1 slice of toast

Cooking time: 5 minutes

Instructions:

1. Toast the whole-wheat bread.
2. Spread the mashed banana on the toast.
3. Top with almond butter and sliced strawberries (optional).
4. Sprinkle with cinnamon if desired.
5. Enjoy a quick and satisfying breakfast with healthy fats and fiber.

Label: Source of healthy fats and vitamin B6, gluten-free option (use gluten-free bread).

# Kale and White Bean Toast

Ingredients:

- 1 slice of whole-wheat bread
- 1/2 cup chopped kale
- 1/4 cup cooked white beans (cannellini or Great Northern)
- 2 tablespoons crumbled ricotta cheese
- 1 tablespoon extra virgin olive oil
- Pinch of salt and pepper

Nutritional Information (per serving):

- Calories: 250
- Fat: 8g (1g saturated)
- Carbs: 30g (5g fiber)
- Protein: 10g
- Calcium: 100mg (10% DV)

Serving size: 1 slice of toast

Cooking time: 10 minutes

**Instructions:**

1. Toast the whole-wheat bread.
2. Sauté the chopped kale in a pan with olive oil for 2-3 minutes until slightly softened.
3. Add the cooked white beans and heat through.
4. Top the toast with the kale and bean mixture, then add crumbled ricotta cheese.
5. Season with salt and pepper to taste.
6. Enjoy a nutrient-dense and flavorful breakfast with protein, fiber, and calcium.

Label: High in protein and fiber, vegetarian, customizable with different herbs and spices.

# Oatmeal with Milk, Nuts, and Dried Fruits

Ingredients:

- 1/2 cup rolled oats
- 1 cup unsweetened almond milk (or dairy milk)
- 1/4 cup sliced almonds
- 1/4 cup chopped dried cranberries
- 1/4 cup chopped dried apricots
- 1 tablespoon honey (optional)
- Pinch of cinnamon

Nutritional Information (per serving):

- Calories: 300
- Fat: 8g (1g saturated)
- Carbs: 40g (5g fiber)
- Protein: 8g
- Calcium: 200mg (20% DV)

Serving size: 1 bowl

Cooking time: 5 minutes

Instructions:

1. In a saucepan, bring the almond milk to a boil. Add the rolled oats and cook for 5 minutes, stirring occasionally, until thickened.
2. Remove from heat and stir in the chopped nuts, dried fruits, honey (optional), and cinnamon.
3. Enjoy a warm and comforting breakfast with whole grains, healthy fats, and vitamins.

Label: Plant-based option (use plant-based milk), vegan (skip honey), fiber-rich and satisfying.

# Baked Egg and Cheese Cups

**Ingredients:**

- 4 eggs
- 1/4 cup shredded cheddar cheese
- 1/4 cup chopped spinach
- Pinch of salt and pepper
- Paprika (optional)

**Nutritional Information (per cup):**

- Calories: 150
- Fat: 10g (5g saturated)
- Carbs: 1g (0g fiber)
- Protein: 12g
- Calcium: 150mg (15% DV)

Serving size: 1 ramekin

Cooking time: 15 minutes

## Instructions:

1. Preheat the oven to 350°F (175°C).
2. Grease 4 ramekins with cooking spray.
3. Crack an egg into each ramekin.
4. Top each egg with shredded cheese, spinach, salt, and pepper.
5. Sprinkle with paprika if desired.
6. Bake for 12-15 minutes, or until the egg whites are set and the yolks are cooked to your liking.
7. Enjoy a protein-packed and versatile breakfast option with vegetables and healthy fats.

Label: Gluten-free, customizable with different vegetables and herbs, perfect for meal prep.

# Panna Cotta with Blueberry, Prune Compote, and Cinnamon

Ingredients:

- Panna Cotta:
    - 2 cups heavy cream
    - 1/2 cup milk (low-fat or unsweetened almond milk option)
    - 1/4 cup sugar
    - 1 vanilla bean, split and scraped
    - 4 sheets (6 grams) gelatin sheets

- Blueberry, Prune Compote:
    - 1 cup fresh blueberries
    - 1/2 cup pitted prunes, chopped
    - 1/4 cup water
    - 1 tablespoon honey
    - 1/4 teaspoon ground cinnamon

Nutritional Information (per serving):

- Calories: 350
- Fat: 20g (10g saturated)
- Carbs: 35g (3g fiber)
- Protein: 8g
- Calcium: 200mg (20% DV)

Serving size: 1 individual panna cotta with compote

Cooking time: 2 hours (mostly chilling time)

Instructions:

1.  Panna Cotta:
    - Pour cream and milk into a saucepan. Add sugar, vanilla bean pod, and seeds, and stir to dissolve sugar.
    - Heat over medium heat until simmering, then remove from heat and cover. Let steep for 30 minutes.
    - While the milk mixture steeps, soak gelatin sheets in cold water for 5-10 minutes until softened.
    - Strain the steeped milk mixture back into the saucepan and gently stir in the softened gelatin sheets until dissolved.
    - Divide the mixture among 4 ramekins or small serving glasses. Refrigerate for at least 2 hours, or until firm.

2. Blueberry, Prune Compote:
    - While panna cotta sets, combine blueberries, prunes, water, honey, and cinnamon in a saucepan.
    - Bring to a simmer over medium heat and cook for 5-7 minutes, stirring occasionally, until prunes are softened and the compote thickens slightly.
    - Let cool slightly before serving on top of the chilled panna cotta.

Label: High in calcium, antioxidant-rich, customizable with different fruits and toppings, gluten-free option (use almond milk).

# Orange and Almond Cake

Ingredients:

- 1 1/2 cups all-purpose flour
- 1/2 cup almond flour
- 1 teaspoon baking powder
- 1/2 teaspoon baking soda
- 1/4 teaspoon salt
- 1/2 cup unsalted butter, softened
- 1 cup granulated sugar
- 2 large eggs
- 1/2 cup freshly squeezed orange juice
- 1/4 cup plain yogurt (low-fat or Greek yogurt option)
- 1 teaspoon vanilla extract
- 1/2 cup chopped almonds (optional)

Nutritional Information (per slice):

- Calories: 250
- Fat: 12g (2g saturated)
- Carbs: 30g (2g fiber)
- Protein: 5g
- Calcium: 50mg (5% DV)

Serving size: 12 slices

Cooking time: 45 minutes

Instructions:

1. Preheat the oven to 350°F/175°C. Butter and flour in a 9x5 loaf pan.

2. Whisk together the dry ingredients (flour, baking powder, baking soda, and salt) in a medium mixing basin.

3. Cream together the butter and sugar in a large mixing mixer until light and creamy. One at a time beat in the eggs, then whisk in the orange juice, yogurt, and vanilla extract.

4. Add the dry ingredients to the liquid components gradually, mixing until just mixed. If using, fold in the chopped almonds.

5. Smooth the top of the batter into the prepared pan.

6. Preheat the oven to 45-50 minutes, or until a toothpick inserted into the middle comes out clean.

7. Allow to cool for 10 minutes in the pan before transferring to a wire rack to cool fully.

Label: High in fiber, vitamin C, and healthy fats, gluten-free option (use all almond flour), dairy-free option (use plant-based yogurt and milk alternative).

# Lunch Recipes

## Vegetarian Pita

Ingredients:

- 1 whole wheat pita bread
- 1/2 cup hummus
- 1/4 cup chopped cucumber
- 1/4 cup chopped red onion
- 1/4 cup chopped red bell pepper
- 1/4 cup crumbled feta cheese
- 1 tablespoon chopped fresh parsley
- Pinch of salt and pepper

Nutritional Information (per pita):

- Calories: 300
- Fat: 10g (3g saturated)
- Carbs: 40g (5g fiber)
- Protein: 15g
- Calcium: 200mg (20% DV)

Serving size: 1 pita

Cooking time: 5 minutes

**Instructions:**

1. Spread hummus evenly on the pita bread.
2. Top with chopped cucumber, red onion, and red bell pepper.
3. Crumble feta cheese over the vegetables.
4. Sprinkle with parsley, salt, and pepper to taste.
5. Fold the pita in half and enjoy a portable and protein-packed lunch with fiber and calcium.

Label: Vegetarian, high in fiber, customizable with different vegetables and toppings.

# Turkey-Roquefort Salad

**Ingredients:**

- 3 ounces sliced turkey breast
- 2 cups mixed greens
- 1/2 cup chopped romaine lettuce
- 1/4 cup sliced green grapes
- 1/4 cup crumbled blue cheese (Roquefort or Gorgonzola)
- 2 tablespoons balsamic vinaigrette dressing
- Pinch of salt and pepper

**Nutritional Information (per salad):**

- Calories: 350
- Fat: 15g (5g saturated)
- Carbs: 15g (3g fiber)
- Protein: 30g
- Calcium: 150mg (15% DV)

Serving size: 1 salad

Cooking time: 10 minutes

## Instructions:

1. Toss the mixed greens, romaine lettuce, turkey breast, and grapes in a bowl.
2. Crumble the blue cheese over the salad.
3. Drizzle with balsamic vinaigrette dressing and toss to coat.
4. Season with salt and pepper to taste.
5. Enjoy a flavorful and protein-rich salad with healthy fats and vitamins.

Label: Gluten-free, dairy-free option (omit blue cheese), a good source of iron and antioxidants.

# Quinoa, Shrimp, and Broccoli Salad

Ingredients:

- 1 cup cooked quinoa
- 1/2 pound cooked shrimp, peeled and deveined
- 1 cup steamed broccoli florets
- 1/4 cup chopped red onion
- 1/4 cup chopped celery
- 2 tablespoons lemon juice
- 1 tablespoon olive oil
- Pinch of salt and pepper

Nutritional Information (per serving):

- Calories: 300
- Fat: 8g (1g saturated)
- Carbs: 35g (5g fiber)
- Protein: 25g
- Calcium: 50mg (5% DV)

Serving size: 1 salad

Cooking time: 20 minutes (includes cooking time for quinoa and shrimp)

Instructions:

1. Combine the cooked quinoa, shrimp, broccoli florets, red onion, and celery in a bowl.
2. In a small mixing bowl, combine the lemon juice and olive oil.
3. Toss the salad with the dressing to coat.
4. Season with salt and pepper to taste.
5. Enjoy a refreshing and nutrient-packed salad with whole grains, protein, and vegetables.

Label: Gluten-free, high in fiber and protein, low-fat option (use less olive oil), great for meal prep.

# Spinach Salad with Herbs, Goat Cheese, and Cashews

Ingredients:

- 4 cups baby spinach
- 1/2 cup chopped fresh herbs (mix of parsley, basil, chives, and mint)
- 1/4 cup crumbled goat cheese
- 1/4 cup roasted and chopped cashews
- 2 tablespoons extra virgin olive oil
- 1 tablespoon lemon juice
- Pinch of salt and pepper

**Nutritional Information (per serving):**

- Calories: 350
- Fat: 18g (4g saturated)
- Carbs: 8g (2g fiber)
- Protein: 12g
- Calcium: 200mg (20% DV)

Serving size: 1 salad

Cooking time: 5 minutes

**Instructions:**

1. Toss the spinach and chopped herbs in a bowl.
2. Crumble goat cheese over the salad.
3. Sprinkle with roasted cashews.
4. In a small mixing bowl, combine the olive oil, lemon juice, salt, and pepper.
5. Toss the salad with the dressing to coat it.
6. Enjoy a flavorful and nutrient-rich salad with protein, healthy fats, and vitamins.

Label: High in protein and antioxidants, vegetarian, customizable with different greens and toppings.

# Greek Yogurt Parfait with Granola and Berries

**Ingredients:**

- 1 cup plain Greek yogurt (2% fat)
- 1/4 cup granola
- 1/2 cup mixed berries (fresh or frozen)
- 1 tablespoon honey (optional)
- Pinch of cinnamon

**Nutritional Information (per parfait):**

- Calories: 300
- Fat: 5g (2g saturated)
- Carbs: 30g (5g fiber)
- Protein: 20g
- Calcium: 300mg (30% DV)

Serving size: 1 parfait

Cooking time: 5 minutes

Instructions:

1. Layer the Greek yogurt, granola, and berries in a glass or parfait dish.
2. Drizzle with honey if desired and sprinkle with cinnamon.
3. Enjoy a refreshing and protein-packed snack or light lunch with probiotics, fiber, and vitamins.

Label: High in protein and calcium, good source of probiotics, vegan option (use plant-based yogurt).

# Cheese and Tomato Sandwich

Ingredients:

- 2 slices whole-wheat bread
- 2 slices tomato
- 2 slices cheddar cheese
- 1 tablespoon mayonnaise (optional)
- 1/4 teaspoon Dijon mustard (optional)
- Lettuce and spinach (optional)

Nutritional Information (per sandwich):

- Calories: 350
- Fat: 15g (5g saturated)
- Carbs: 40g (5g fiber)
- Protein: 15g
- Calcium: 300mg (30% DV)

Serving size: 1 sandwich

Cooking time: 5 minutes

Instructions:

1. Toast the bread if desired.
2. Spread mayonnaise or Dijon mustard on one slice of bread (optional).
3. Layer cheese and tomato slices on the bread.
4. Add lettuce and spinach if desired.
5. Top with the other slice of bread and enjoy a simple and satisfying lunch with calcium, fiber, and healthy fats.

Label: Customizable with different cheeses and vegetables, gluten-free option (use gluten-free bread).

# Creamy Mushroom and Spinach Pasta

## Ingredients:

- 8 ounces whole-wheat pasta (penne, fusilli, or your favorite)
- 1 tablespoon olive oil
- 1/2 onion, chopped
- 4 ounces mushrooms, sliced
- 2 cloves garlic, minced
- 1/2 cup low-fat milk
- 1/4 cup ricotta cheese
- 1/4 cup chopped fresh spinach
- 1/4 cup grated Parmesan cheese
- Pinch of salt and pepper
- Fresh herbs (optional, such as basil or parsley)

## Nutritional Information (per serving):

- Calories: 350
- Fat: 8g (2g saturated)
- Carbs: 45g (6g fiber)
- Protein: 15g
- Calcium: 200mg (20% DV)

Serving size: 1 cup

Cooking time: 20 minutes

Instructions:

1. Cook the pasta according to package instructions.
2. While pasta cooks, heat olive oil in a pan over medium heat. Cook until the onion is softened, approximately 5 minutes.
3. Add mushrooms and garlic, and cook until browned, about 5 minutes more.
4. Stir in milk, ricotta cheese, and spinach. Season with salt and pepper.
5. Once the pasta is cooked, drain and add to the pan with the sauce. Toss to combine.
6. Serve topped with Parmesan cheese and fresh herbs if desired.

Label: High in fiber, vegetarian, customizable with different vegetables and toppings.

# Roasted Vegetable and Hummus Wrap

Ingredients:

- 2 whole wheat tortillas
- 1/2 cup mixed roasted vegetables (bell peppers, zucchini, onions, etc.)
- 1/4 cup hummus
- 1/4 cup crumbled feta cheese
- 1/4 cup romaine lettuce, chopped
- Fresh herbs (optional)

Nutritional Information (per wrap):

- Calories: 300
- Fat: 8g (2g saturated)
- Carbs: 40g (5g fiber)
- Protein: 12g
- Calcium: 200mg (20% DV)

Serving size: 1 wrap

Cooking time: 20 minutes (includes roasting time)

Instructions:

1. Preheat the oven to 400°F (200°C). Toss vegetables with olive oil and spices of your choice, then spread on a baking sheet. Roast for 20 minutes, or until the potatoes are soft.
2. Spread hummus on a tortilla. Top with roasted vegetables, feta cheese, romaine lettuce, and fresh herbs.
3. Roll up the tortilla and enjoy a portable and flavorful lunch or dinner.

Label: Vegan option (omit feta cheese), gluten-free option (use gluten-free tortillas), high in antioxidants and fiber.

# Tuna and White Bean Salad

**Ingredients:**

- 1 can (5 oz) tuna, drained and flaked
- 1 cup cooked white beans (cannellini or chickpeas)
- 1/2 cup chopped cucumber
- 1/4 cup chopped red onion
- 1/4 cup chopped celery
- 2 tablespoons lemon juice
- 1 tablespoon olive oil
- 1/4 teaspoon dried dill
- Pinch of salt and pepper

**Nutritional Information (per serving):**

- Calories: 300
- Fat: 5g (1g saturated)
- Carbs: 30g (5g fiber)
- Protein: 25g
- Calcium: 50mg (5% DV)

Serving size: 1 cup

Cooking time: 10 minutes

Instructions:

1. Combine tuna, beans, cucumber, red onion, and celery in a bowl.
2. Whisk together lemon juice, olive oil, dill, salt, and pepper in a small bowl.
3. Toss the salad with the dressing to coat.
4. Serve on a bed of lettuce or enjoy as a snack or light dinner.

Label: High in protein and fiber, gluten-free, customizable with different vegetables and spices.

# Dinner Recipes

## Paprika Chicken with Prunes and Breadcrumb Crust

Ingredients:

- 4 boneless, skinless chicken breasts (approximately 6 ounces each)
- 1/2 teaspoon salt
- 1/4 teaspoon black pepper
- 1/4 teaspoon paprika
- 1/4 teaspoon garlic powder
- 1/2 cup sliced prunes
- 1/4 cup chopped walnuts
- 1/4 cup dry breadcrumbs
- 1/4 cup grated Parmesan cheese
- 2 tablespoons olive oil

Nutritional Information (per serving):

- Calories: 350
- Fat: 15g (2g saturated)
- Carbs: 25g (3g fiber)
- Protein: 35g
- Calcium: 50mg (5% DV)

Serving size: 1 chicken breast

Cooking time: 25 minutes

Instructions:

1. Preheat the oven to 400°F (200°C).
2. Season chicken breasts with salt, pepper, paprika, and garlic powder.
3. Sauté the sliced prunes in olive oil for 2-3 minutes until softened.
4. Combine chopped walnuts, breadcrumbs, Parmesan cheese, and remaining olive oil in a bowl.
5. Spread the prune mixture over the chicken breasts, then top with the breadcrumb crust.
6. Place on a baking sheet and bake for 20-25 minutes, or until chicken is cooked through and the crust is golden brown.

Label: High in protein, gluten-free option (use gluten-free breadcrumbs), good source of iron and antioxidants.

# Beetroot Soup with Prune Dumplings

## Ingredients:

- 4 medium beets, peeled and chopped
- 1 onion, chopped
- 2 cloves garlic, minced
- 4 cups vegetable broth
- 1/4 cup chopped prunes
- 1/4 cup chopped walnuts
- 1/4 cup whole-wheat flour
- 1/4 teaspoon thyme
- Pinch of salt and pepper

## Nutritional Information (per serving):

- Calories: 250
- Fat: 5g (1g saturated)
- Carbs: 30g (5g fiber)
- Protein: 5g
- Calcium: 30mg (3% DV)

Serving size: 1 bowl

Cooking time: 30 minutes

Instructions:

1. Sauté onion and garlic in a pot with olive oil.
2. Add beets and vegetable broth, then bring to a boil. Reduce heat and simmer for 20 minutes, or until beets are tender.
3. Using an immersion blender or in batches in a conventional blender, puree the soup.
4. While the soup is simmering, make a dough using the prunes, walnuts, flour, thyme, salt, and pepper.
5. Make little dumplings out of the dough and put them into the boiling broth. Cook for 5-7 minutes, or until the dumplings are tender.
6. Serve the soup warm with a dollop of yogurt or plant-based yogurt if desired.

Label: Vegan option (omit yogurt), high in fiber and antioxidants, customizable with different herbs and spices.

# Veal Cordon Bleu

**Ingredients:**

- 4 thin veal cutlets (about 4 oz each)
- 4 slices low-fat ham
- 4 slices Swiss cheese (reduced-fat option)
- 1/4 cup whole-wheat flour
- 1 egg, beaten
- 1/2 cup panko breadcrumbs
- 1 teaspoon paprika
- 1/4 teaspoon garlic powder
- Pinch of salt and pepper
- 2 tablespoons olive oil or grapeseed oil

**Nutritional Information (per serving):**

- Calories: 350
- Fat: 15g (3g saturated)
- Carbs: 20g (2g fiber)
- Protein: 35g
- Calcium: 200mg (20% DV)

Serving size: 1 veal cordon bleu

Cooking time: 20 minutes

**Instructions:**

1. Pound the veal cutlets thin between two pieces of plastic wrap, if needed. Season with salt and pepper.
2. Place a piece of ham and a slice of cheese on top of each cutlet. Roll up the cutlet and secure it with toothpicks.
3. Dredge the rolled cutlets in flour, then in beaten egg, and finally in the panko breadcrumbs mixed with paprika and garlic powder.
4. Air fryer option: Preheat your air fryer to 400°F (200°C). Lightly spray the breaded cutlets with cooking spray. Place them in the air fryer basket and cook for 10-12 minutes per side or until golden brown and cooked through.
5. Pan option: Heat oil in a pan over medium heat. Carefully place the breaded cutlets in the pan and cook for 3-4 minutes per side or until golden brown and cooked through.
6. Once cooked, remove the cutlets from the pan or air fryer and let them rest for a few minutes before serving.

Labels: High in protein, gluten-free option (use gluten-free flour and breadcrumbs), customizable with different cheeses and vegetables.

# Spinach and Ricotta Parcels

## Ingredients:

- 1 sheet frozen puff pastry, thawed
- 10 ounces fresh spinach, blanched and squeezed dry
- 1/2 cup ricotta cheese
- 1/4 cup grated Parmesan cheese
- 1 egg yolk, beaten
- 1 tablespoon olive oil
- Pinch of salt and pepper

## Nutritional Information (per parcel):

- Calories: 250
- Fat: 12g (3g saturated)
- Carbs: 20g (1g fiber)
- Protein: 10g
- Calcium: 200mg (20% DV)

Serving size: 4 parcels

Cooking time: 25 minutes

Instructions:

1.  Preheat the oven to 400°F (200°C). Line a baking sheet with parchment paper.
2.  Unfold the puff pastry sheet and cut it into 4 squares.
3.  Combine spinach, ricotta cheese, Parmesan cheese, salt, and pepper in a bowl.
4.  Spoon the ricotta mixture onto the center of each pastry square. Brush the edges with egg yolk.
5.  Fold the pastry diagonally into triangles, pressing the edges closed with a fork.
6.  Brush the tops of the parcels with the remaining egg yolk.
7.  Bake for 20 to 25 minutes or until golden brown and puffy.
8.  Serve warm as a light appetizer or snack.

Label: High in protein and calcium, vegetarian, customizable with different cheeses and herbs.

# Spicy Sardine and Parmesan Fritters

Ingredients:

- 1 can (5 oz) sardines in oil, drained
- 1/2 cup mashed potatoes
- 1/4 cup chopped red onion
- 1/4 cup chopped red bell pepper
- 1 tablespoon chopped fresh parsley
- 1 tablespoon chopped fresh cilantro
- 1/2 teaspoon chili powder
- 1/4 teaspoon smoked paprika
- Pinch of salt and pepper
- 1/4 cup all-purpose flour
- 2 tablespoons vegetable oil

Nutritional Information (per fritter):

- Calories: 150
- Fat: 8g (1g saturated)
- Carbs: 15g (1g fiber)
- Protein: 10g
- Calcium: 80mg (8% DV)

Serving size: 8 fritters

Cooking time: 15 minutes

**Instructions:**

1. In a bowl, mash the sardines with a fork.
2. Add mashed potatoes, red onion, red bell pepper, parsley, cilantro, chili powder, paprika, salt, and pepper. Stir to combine.
3. Mix in the flour until just incorporated.
4. In a frying pan over medium heat, heat the oil.
5. Drop tablespoonfuls of the mixture into the oil and cook for 2-3 minutes per side or until golden brown and cooked through.
6. Drain on paper towels and serve with a lemon wedge or tartar sauce.

Label: High in protein and healthy fats, gluten-free option (use gluten-free flour), a good source of omega-3 fatty acids.

# Quiche Lorraine

Ingredients:

- 1 pie crust (homemade or store-bought)
- 6 slices bacon, cooked and chopped
- 1/2 cup chopped onion
- 1/4 cup chopped leeks
- 2 cloves garlic, minced
- 4 eggs
- 1 cup milk (low-fat or unsweetened almond milk)
- 1/2 cup shredded Gruyère cheese
- 1/4 cup shredded Swiss cheese
- 1/4 teaspoon nutmeg
- Pinch of salt and pepper

Nutritional Information (per slice):

- Calories: 300
- Fat: 15g (5g saturated)
- Carbs: 20g (2g fiber)
- Protein: 15g
- Calcium: 250mg (25% DV)

Serving size: 6 slices

Cooking time: 40 minutes

**Instructions:**

1. Preheat the oven to 375°F (190°C). Blind bake the pie crust according to package instructions, or poke the bottom with a fork and bake for 10 minutes.
2. While the crust cooks, sauté the bacon, onion, leeks, and garlic in a pan until softened.
3. Whisk together the eggs, milk, Gruyère cheese, Swiss cheese, nutmeg, salt, and pepper in a bowl.
4. Pour the egg mixture into the pre-baked pie crust, then scatter the bacon and sautéed vegetables on top.
5. Bake for 25-30 minutes, or until the filling is firm and golden brown.

6. Allow it to cool for at least 10 minutes before slicing and serving.

# Scrambled-Egg Stir-Fry

Ingredients:

- 2 eggs
- 1 tablespoon olive oil
- 1/2 cup chopped bell peppers (mix of colors)
- 1/4 cup chopped onion
- 1/4 cup chopped broccoli florets
- 1 tablespoon chopped fresh basil
- Pinch of salt and pepper
- Optional: 1/4 cup cooked brown rice or quinoa

Nutritional Information (per serving):

- Calories: 250
- Fat: 8g (2g saturated)
- Carbs: 8g (1g fiber)
- Protein: 18g
- Calcium: 50mg (5% DV)

Serving size: 1 stir-fry bowl

Cooking time: 10 minutes

**Instructions:**

1. In a mixing dish, combine the eggs, salt, and pepper.
2. Heat olive oil in a pan or wok over medium heat. Add bell peppers and onion, and cook until softened about 5 minutes.
3. Add broccoli and cook for another 2-3 minutes.
4. Push the vegetables to one side of the pan and pour in the egg mixture. Scramble eggs until cooked through.
5. Stir in the basil and serve over cooked brown rice or quinoa if desired.

Label: High in protein, customizable with different vegetables and herbs, gluten-free option (omit rice or quinoa).

# Salmon, Kale, and Turnip Greens Soup

Ingredients:

- 1 tablespoon olive oil
- 1 onion, chopped
- 2 cloves garlic, minced
- 4 cups vegetable broth
- 2 stalks celery, chopped
- 1 cup chopped kale
- 1 cup chopped turnip greens
- 1 can (14.5 oz) salmon, drained and flaked
- 1/2 cup plain Greek yogurt (2% fat)
- Pinch of salt and pepper
- Fresh herbs (optional)

Nutritional Information (per serving):

- Calories: 300
- Fat: 8g (2g saturated)
- Carbs: 15g (3g fiber)
- Protein: 30g
- Calcium: 200mg (20% DV)

Serving size: 1 bowl

Cooking time: 25 minutes

**Instructions:**

1. In a medium-sized saucepan, heat the olive oil. Cook until the onion is softened, approximately 5 minutes.
2. Cook for another minute after adding the garlic.
3. Bring to a boil with the veggie broth. Add celery, kale, and turnip greens.
4. Reduce heat and simmer for 10 minutes, or until greens are tender.
5. Add flaked salmon and cook for an additional 2-3 minutes.
6. Stir in Greek yogurt, salt, and pepper.
7. Serve hot with fresh herbs like dill or parsley if desired.

Label: High in protein and calcium, good source of vitamins and minerals, vegan option (use plant-based yogurt).

# Omelet with Cheddar Cheese, Sautéed Greens, and Salmon

**Ingredients:**

- 2 eggs
- 1 tablespoon milk
- Pinch of salt and pepper
- 1 tablespoon butter
- 1/2 cup chopped spinach or arugula
- 1/4 cup crumbled cheddar cheese
- 1 cooked salmon fillet, flaked

**Nutritional Information (per serving):**

- Calories: 350
- Fat: 15g (5g saturated)
- Carbs: 5g (1g fiber)
- Protein: 25g
- Calcium: 250mg (25% DV)

Serving size: 1 omelet

Cooking time: 10 minutes

**Instructions:**

1. Whisk eggs, milk, salt, and pepper in a bowl.
2. Melt butter in a pan over medium heat. Pour in the egg mixture and cook until the sides are almost set.
3. Sprinkle it with spinach or arugula and cheese. Fold the omelet in half.
4. Add flaked salmon to the center of the omelet and fold again.
5. Serve hot with a side of avocado or fruit salad.

Label: High in protein and calcium, low-carb option, customizable with different cheeses and fillings.

# Broccoli and Cheese Frittata

Ingredients:

- 8 eggs
- 1/2 cup milk (low-fat or unsweetened almond milk)
- 1/4 cup grated Parmesan cheese
- 1 tablespoon olive oil
- 2 cups chopped broccoli florets
- 1/2 cup chopped onion
- 1/4 cup chopped red bell pepper (optional)
- 1/2 cup shredded cheddar cheese
- Pinch of salt and pepper
- Fresh herbs (optional)

Nutritional Information (per serving):

- Calories: 300
- Fat: 12g (3g saturated)
- Carbs: 15g (2g fiber)
- Protein: 20g
- Calcium: 300mg (30% DV)

Serving size: 1 wedge

Cooking time: 30 minutes

Instructions:

1. Preheat the oven to 400°F (200°C). Grease a 10-inch oven-safe skillet.
2. Whisk eggs, milk, Parmesan cheese, salt, and pepper in a bowl.
3. Heat olive oil in the skillet over medium heat. Add onion and bell pepper (if using) and cook until softened, about 5 minutes.
4. Add broccoli and cook for another 3-4 minutes, until slightly tender.
5. Pour the egg mixture into the skillet and sprinkle with cheddar cheese.
6. Bake for 20-25 minutes, or until the frittata is set and golden brown.
7. Let cool slightly and serve warm, garnished with fresh herbs if desired.

Label: High in protein and calcium, gluten-free option (omit crust), customizable with different vegetables and cheeses.

# Cauliflower and Cheese Casserole

Ingredients:

- 1 head cauliflower, cut into florets
- 1 tablespoon olive oil
- 1/2 cup chopped onion
- 2 cloves garlic, minced
- 2 cups grated cheddar cheese (divided)
- 1/2 cup shredded Parmesan cheese
- 1/4 cup all-purpose flour (gluten-free option available)
- 2 cups milk (low-fat or unsweetened almond milk)
- 1/2 teaspoon salt
- 1/4 teaspoon black pepper
- Pinch of paprika

Nutritional Information (per serving):

- Calories: 350
- Fat: 20g (8g saturated)
- Carbs: 25g (3g fiber)
- Protein: 20g
- Calcium: 400mg (40% DV)

Serving size: 1/6 casserole dish

Cooking time: 45 minutes

Instructions:

1. Preheat the oven to 375°F (190°C). Grease a 9x13-inch baking dish.
2. Steam or boil cauliflower until tender. Drain and mash coarsely.
3. In a skillet over medium heat, heat the olive oil. Cook until the onion is softened, approximately 5 minutes.
4. Add garlic and cook for another minute.
5. Stir in 1 cup cheddar cheese, Parmesan cheese, flour, salt, pepper, and paprika.
6. Slowly whisk in milk until a smooth sauce forms.
7. Combine sauce with mashed cauliflower and pour into the prepared baking dish.
8. Sprinkle it with the remaining cheddar cheese.
9. Bake for 30-35 minutes, or until the casserole is bubbly and golden brown.

Label: High in calcium and fiber, vegetarian option, gluten-free option (use gluten-free flour).

# Chicken and Broccoli Alfredo

**Ingredients:**

- 1 tablespoon olive oil
- 1 boneless, skinless chicken breast, sliced
- 2 cups broccoli florets
- 1/2 cup low-fat ricotta cheese
- 1/4 cup grated Parmesan cheese
- 1/4 cup milk (low-fat or unsweetened almond milk)
- 1 teaspoon Dijon mustard
- Pinch of salt and pepper
- Whole-wheat pasta or zoodles (spiralized zucchini)

**Nutritional Information (per serving):**

- Calories: 400
- Fat: 12g (2g saturated)
- Carbs: 40g (5g fiber)
- Protein: 35g
- Calcium: 250mg (25% DV)

Serving size: 1 plate

Cooking time: 20 minutes

Instructions:

1.  Cook the pasta: Boil whole-wheat pasta according to package instructions. If opting for zoodles, skip this step and prepare your zucchini by spiralizing it with a spiralizer or julienne peeler.

2.  Prepare the chicken and broccoli: While the pasta is cooking, heat the olive oil in a skillet over medium heat. Add the sliced chicken and cook until golden brown and cooked through about 5-7 minutes. Set cooked chicken aside.

3.  Steam the broccoli: Add the broccoli florets to a steamer basket and steam for 3-4 minutes or until slightly tender-crisp. This will help retain nutrients and maintain a vibrant texture.

4.  Make the sauce: In a separate bowl, whisk together the ricotta cheese, Parmesan cheese, milk, Dijon mustard, salt, and pepper. This creamy sauce will be the base for our Alfredo.

5.  Combine and finish: Once the pasta or zoodles are cooked and the chicken and

broccoli are ready, drain the pasta and add it to the pan with the chicken and broccoli.

6.  Pour the ricotta cheese mixture over the pasta and vegetables, and toss to combine. Gently heat through for 1-2 minutes, allowing the sauce to coat everything evenly.

7.  Serve and enjoy: Serve immediately topped with additional freshly grated Parmesan cheese if desired. Pair this lighter and osteoporotically-friendly take on Alfredo with a side salad for a balanced and nutritious meal.

# Conclusion

You have reached the end of this book, but not the end of your journey to better bone health. By following the osteoporosis diet, you have taken a powerful step towards preventing and treating this condition that affects millions of people worldwide. But eating well is not enough. You also need to exercise regularly, avoid smoking and alcohol, and consult your doctor about any medications or supplements that may affect your bones. Remember, osteoporosis is not a death sentence. It is a manageable condition that can be improved with the right lifestyle choices. We hope you enjoyed the recipes in this book and found them easy to prepare and delicious to eat. We also hope you learned something new about the benefits of calcium, vitamin D, and other nutrients for your bones. Feel free to experiment with the ingredients and create your variations of the dishes. The most important thing is to have fun and enjoy your food!

Thank you for choosing this book and trusting us with your health. We wish you all the best and hope to hear from you soon. Please leave us a review and let us know what you think of the book and the recipes. Your feedback is valuable and appreciated. Until next time, happy cooking and healthy bones!

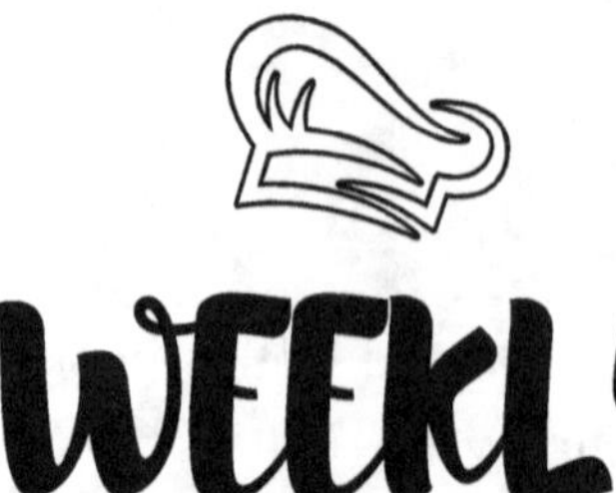

# WEEKLY MEAL PLANNER

# WEEKLY MEAL PLANNER

| | | |
|---|---|---|
| **SUNDAY** | BREAKFAST | |
| | LUNCH | |
| | DINNER | |
| **MONDAY** | BREAKFAST | |
| | LUNCH | |
| | DINNER | |
| **TUESDAY** | BREAKFAST | |
| | LUNCH | |
| | DINNER | |
| **WEDNESDAY** | BREAKFAST | |
| | LUNCH | |
| | DINNER | |
| **THURSDAY** | BREAKFAST | |
| | LUNCH | |
| | DINNER | |
| **FRIDAY** | BREAKFAST | |
| | LUNCH | |
| | DINNER | |
| **SATURDAY** | BREAKFAST | |
| | LUNCH | |
| | DINNER | |

**GROCERY LIST**

**SNACKS**

# WEEKLY MEAL PLANNER

| | | |
|---|---|---|
| **SUNDAY** | BREAKFAST | |
| | LUNCH | |
| | DINNER | |
| **MONDAY** | BREAKFAST | |
| | LUNCH | |
| | DINNER | |
| **TUESDAY** | BREAKFAST | |
| | LUNCH | |
| | DINNER | |
| **WEDNESDAY** | BREAKFAST | |
| | LUNCH | |
| | DINNER | |
| **THURSDAY** | BREAKFAST | |
| | LUNCH | |
| | DINNER | |
| **FRIDAY** | BREAKFAST | |
| | LUNCH | |
| | DINNER | |
| **SATURDAY** | BREAKFAST | |
| | LUNCH | |
| | DINNER | |

**GROCERY LIST**

**SNACKS**

# WEEKLY MEAL PLANNER

| SUNDAY | BREAKFAST | |
| | LUNCH | |
| | DINNER | |

**GROCERY LIST**

| MONDAY | BREAKFAST | |
| | LUNCH | |
| | DINNER | |

| TUESDAY | BREAKFAST | |
| | LUNCH | |
| | DINNER | |

| WEDNESDAY | BREAKFAST | |
| | LUNCH | |
| | DINNER | |

| THURSDAY | BREAKFAST | |
| | LUNCH | |
| | DINNER | |

**SNACKS**

| FRIDAY | BREAKFAST | |
| | LUNCH | |
| | DINNER | |

| SATURDAY | BREAKFAST | |
| | LUNCH | |
| | DINNER | |

# WEEKLY MEAL PLANNER

| | | |
|---|---|---|
| **SUNDAY** | BREAKFAST | |
| | LUNCH | |
| | DINNER | |
| **MONDAY** | BREAKFAST | |
| | LUNCH | |
| | DINNER | |
| **TUESDAY** | BREAKFAST | |
| | LUNCH | |
| | DINNER | |
| **WEDNESDAY** | BREAKFAST | |
| | LUNCH | |
| | DINNER | |
| **THURSDAY** | BREAKFAST | |
| | LUNCH | |
| | DINNER | |
| **FRIDAY** | BREAKFAST | |
| | LUNCH | |
| | DINNER | |
| **SATURDAY** | BREAKFAST | |
| | LUNCH | |
| | DINNER | |

GROCERY LIST

SNACKS

# WEEKLY MEAL PLANNER

| | | |
|---|---|---|
| **SUNDAY** | BREAKFAST | |
| | LUNCH | |
| | DINNER | |
| **MONDAY** | BREAKFAST | |
| | LUNCH | |
| | DINNER | |
| **TUESDAY** | BREAKFAST | |
| | LUNCH | |
| | DINNER | |
| **WEDNESDAY** | BREAKFAST | |
| | LUNCH | |
| | DINNER | |
| **THURSDAY** | BREAKFAST | |
| | LUNCH | |
| | DINNER | |
| **FRIDAY** | BREAKFAST | |
| | LUNCH | |
| | DINNER | |
| **SATURDAY** | BREAKFAST | |
| | LUNCH | |
| | DINNER | |

## GROCERY LIST

## SNACKS

# WEEKLY MEAL PLANNER

| SUNDAY | BREAKFAST | |
| | LUNCH | |
| | DINNER | |

| MONDAY | BREAKFAST | |
| | LUNCH | |
| | DINNER | |

| TUESDAY | BREAKFAST | |
| | LUNCH | |
| | DINNER | |

| WEDNESDAY | BREAKFAST | |
| | LUNCH | |
| | DINNER | |

| THURSDAY | BREAKFAST | |
| | LUNCH | |
| | DINNER | |

| FRIDAY | BREAKFAST | |
| | LUNCH | |
| | DINNER | |

| SATURDAY | BREAKFAST | |
| | LUNCH | |
| | DINNER | |

GROCERY LIST

SNACKS

# WEEKLY MEAL PLANNER

| SUNDAY | BREAKFAST | |
| | LUNCH | |
| | DINNER | |
| MONDAY | BREAKFAST | |
| | LUNCH | |
| | DINNER | |
| TUESDAY | BREAKFAST | |
| | LUNCH | |
| | DINNER | |
| WEDNESDAY | BREAKFAST | |
| | LUNCH | |
| | DINNER | |
| THURSDAY | BREAKFAST | |
| | LUNCH | |
| | DINNER | |
| FRIDAY | BREAKFAST | |
| | LUNCH | |
| | DINNER | |
| SATURDAY | BREAKFAST | |
| | LUNCH | |
| | DINNER | |

**GROCERY LIST**

**SNACKS**

# WEEKLY MEAL PLANNER

| | | |
|---|---|---|
| **SUNDAY** | BREAKFAST | |
| | LUNCH | |
| | DINNER | |
| **MONDAY** | BREAKFAST | |
| | LUNCH | |
| | DINNER | |
| **TUESDAY** | BREAKFAST | |
| | LUNCH | |
| | DINNER | |
| **WEDNESDAY** | BREAKFAST | |
| | LUNCH | |
| | DINNER | |
| **THURSDAY** | BREAKFAST | |
| | LUNCH | |
| | DINNER | |
| **FRIDAY** | BREAKFAST | |
| | LUNCH | |
| | DINNER | |
| **SATURDAY** | BREAKFAST | |
| | LUNCH | |
| | DINNER | |

**GROCERY LIST**

**SNACKS**

# WEEKLY MEAL PLANNER

| | | |
|---|---|---|
| **SUNDAY** | BREAKFAST | |
| | LUNCH | |
| | DINNER | |
| **MONDAY** | BREAKFAST | |
| | LUNCH | |
| | DINNER | |
| **TUESDAY** | BREAKFAST | |
| | LUNCH | |
| | DINNER | |
| **WEDNESDAY** | BREAKFAST | |
| | LUNCH | |
| | DINNER | |
| **THURSDAY** | BREAKFAST | |
| | LUNCH | |
| | DINNER | |
| **FRIDAY** | BREAKFAST | |
| | LUNCH | |
| | DINNER | |
| **SATURDAY** | BREAKFAST | |
| | LUNCH | |
| | DINNER | |

GROCERY LIST

SNACKS

# WEEKLY MEAL PLANNER

| | | |
|---|---|---|
| **SUNDAY** | BREAKFAST | |
| | LUNCH | |
| | DINNER | |
| **MONDAY** | BREAKFAST | |
| | LUNCH | |
| | DINNER | |
| **TUESDAY** | BREAKFAST | |
| | LUNCH | |
| | DINNER | |
| **WEDNESDAY** | BREAKFAST | |
| | LUNCH | |
| | DINNER | |
| **THURSDAY** | BREAKFAST | |
| | LUNCH | |
| | DINNER | |
| **FRIDAY** | BREAKFAST | |
| | LUNCH | |
| | DINNER | |
| **SATURDAY** | BREAKFAST | |
| | LUNCH | |
| | DINNER | |

## GROCERY LIST

## SNACKS

# WEEKLY MEAL PLANNER

| | | |
|---|---|---|
| **SUNDAY** | BREAKFAST | |
| | LUNCH | |
| | DINNER | |
| **MONDAY** | BREAKFAST | |
| | LUNCH | |
| | DINNER | |
| **TUESDAY** | BREAKFAST | |
| | LUNCH | |
| | DINNER | |
| **WEDNESDAY** | BREAKFAST | |
| | LUNCH | |
| | DINNER | |
| **THURSDAY** | BREAKFAST | |
| | LUNCH | |
| | DINNER | |
| **FRIDAY** | BREAKFAST | |
| | LUNCH | |
| | DINNER | |
| **SATURDAY** | BREAKFAST | |
| | LUNCH | |
| | DINNER | |

## GROCERY LIST

## SNACKS

# WEEKLY MEAL PLANNER

| SUNDAY | BREAKFAST | |
| | LUNCH | |
| | DINNER | |

| MONDAY | BREAKFAST | |
| | LUNCH | |
| | DINNER | |

| TUESDAY | BREAKFAST | |
| | LUNCH | |
| | DINNER | |

| WEDNESDAY | BREAKFAST | |
| | LUNCH | |
| | DINNER | |

| THURSDAY | BREAKFAST | |
| | LUNCH | |
| | DINNER | |

| FRIDAY | BREAKFAST | |
| | LUNCH | |
| | DINNER | |

| SATURDAY | BREAKFAST | |
| | LUNCH | |
| | DINNER | |

GROCERY LIST

SNACKS